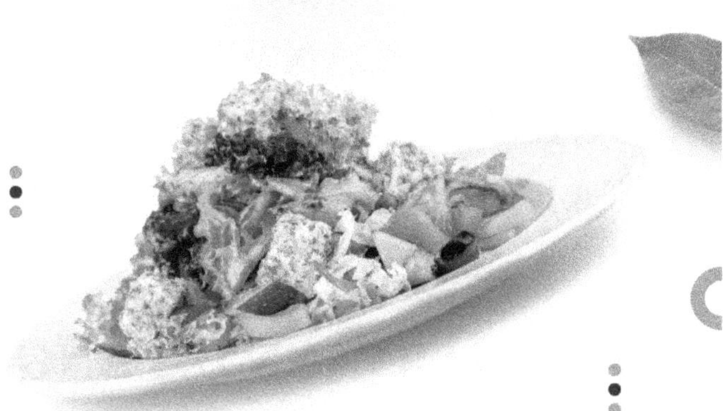

Easy Vegan Meals
To Cook At Home

Let's Live Healthy in a Simple Way

MARYANN D. LANG

EASY VEGAN MEALS TO COOK AT HOME: LET'S LIVE HEALTHY IN A SIMPLE WAY

BY MARYANN D. LANG

COPYRIGHT

© 2024 by **Maryann D. Lang**.

DISCLAIMER

The information contained in this book is for general informational purposes only. While every effort has been made to ensure that the content is accurate and up-to-date, the author makes no representations or warranties of any kind, express or implied, about the completeness, accuracy, reliability, suitability, or availability with respect to the information, products, services, or related graphics contained in this book for any purpose.

Any reliance you place on such information is therefore strictly at your own risk. In no event will the author be liable for any loss or damage including without limitation, indirect or consequential loss or damage, or any loss or damage whatsoever arising from loss of data or profits arising out of, or in connection with, the use of this book.

Every effort is made to keep the book up and running smoothly. However, the author takes no responsibility for, and will not be liable for, the book being temporarily unavailable due to technical issues beyond our control.

ABOUT THE AUTHOR

Maryann D. Lang, a passionate advocate for healthy living, has compiled an exceptional cookbook titled "Easy Vegan Meals to Cook at Home: Let's Live Healthy in a Simple Way." With a focus on simplicity and health, Lang's cookbook offers a delightful array of plant-based recipes that are not only nutritious but also incredibly easy to prepare.Drawing from her own experiences as a vegan home cook, Lang understands the challenges many face when transitioning to a plant-based diet. In her book, she provides a diverse selection of recipes ranging from quick breakfast options to hearty dinners and decadent desserts, ensuring there is something for everyone.What sets Lang's cookbook apart is its emphasis on simplicity. Recognizing that many people lead busy lives, she has carefully crafted recipes that require minimal ingredients and preparation time, making it easy for anyone to whip up delicious vegan meals at home without feeling overwhelmed.Whether you're a seasoned vegan looking for new recipe ideas or someone curious about incorporating more plant-based meals into your diet, "Easy Vegan Meals to Cook at Home" is the perfect companion on your journey to a healthier, more sustainable lifestyle. With Lang's guidance, you'll discover just how easy and delicious vegan cooking can be.

TABLE OF CONTENT

INTRODUCTION

Welcome to Your Deliciously Simple Vegan Journey!

Do you remember when you promised to eat better? It could have been after a checkup, a New Year's vow, or just feeling tired. It was all three for me! Meals were a chore for me because they were full of prepared foods that made me feel tired. After that, I learned about vegan cooking, and everything changed.

To be honest, at first, it seemed really hard to give up meat and cheese. But there's good news: vegan food doesn't have to be bland or dull. It can be bright, fun, and, most importantly, very simple to make at home.

Within these pages, I'm here to guide you on a delicious journey. We'll study the benefits of plant-based eating, from boosting your energy to helping the planet. We'll make a simple vegan pantry, replace common foods with delicious plant-based options, and learn how to quickly make delicious meals. Forget fancy cooking methods and expensive ingredients. This is all about making healthy, tasty meals that fit into your busy life.

Ready to ditch the confusion and accept a world of flavorful, healthy vegan food? Let's ditch the "diet" mentality and unlock the delicious possibilities of your kitchen. Turn the page, and together, we'll start on a journey to a simpler, healthier you!

PART 1: VEGAN STAPLES AND ESSENTIALS - BUILDING YOUR PLANT-BASED KITCHEN

Welcome to the fun world of cooking for vegans! Let's get your kitchen ready for success before we start with some tasty recipes. With a well-stocked pantry, smart ingredient changes, and useful tools, you should be able to make delicious vegan meals without much trouble after reading this.

Stocking Your Pantry: Vegan Ingredients You Must Have

You can think of your kitchen as a treasure chest full of things you need to make great vegan meals. To get you started, here are some significant things:

1. **Whole grains and starches:** These provide sustained energy and come in many delicious types. Have a lot of brown rice, quinoa, oats, couscous, bulgur wheat, and pasta (whole wheat or chickpea works well). Remember to bring bread. Whole-wheat bread, rolls, and wraps can all be used in many ways.

2. **Beans and Lentils:** Beans and lentils are your vegan best friends because they are full of energy and fiber. Canned options are handy, but dried beans are

budget-friendly and offer more cooking control. Look for types like black beans, kidney beans, chickpeas (garbanzo beans), pinto beans, and lentils (green, brown, or red).

3. **Nuts and Seeds:** These tiny nutritional powerhouses offer healthy fats, protein, and a delicious crunch. Almonds, cashews, walnuts, pecans, sunflower seeds, pumpkin seeds, and chia seeds are great picks. Keep raw or roasted nuts in the pantry, and store nut butters like peanut butter or tahini in the fridge for longer shelf life.

4. **Plant-Based Milks:** Dairy options abound! Choose from

soy milk, almond milk, oat milk, coconut milk (great for curries!), or rice milk based on your recipe and taste preference.

5. **Pantry Staples:** These workhorses add depth and flavor to your cooking. Vegetable broth is a must-have for soups, stews, and sauces. Tomato paste adds richness, while spices like cumin, turmeric, chili powder, paprika, garlic powder, and onion powder are taste game-changers. Don't forget salt, pepper, and a good quality olive oil for cooking.

Tips:

- **Buy in bulk: If** you have the space, buying staples like rice, beans, and nuts in bulk can save you money in the long run.
- **Shop seasonally:** Fresh fruits and vegetables are fantastic, but don't forget frozen choices! They're often flash-frozen at peak freshness and are a budget-friendly way to add variety to your meals.
- **Read labels carefully:** Not all vegan claims are made equal. Check for hidden dairy or eggs in packaged goods.

Easy Swaps: Replacing Animal Products with Plant-Powered Alternatives

Making the switch to vegan doesn't mean giving up your favorite meals! Here are some clever changes to keep your taste buds happy:

Meat:

Ground "meat": Lentils, crumbled tempeh, chopped walnuts, or textured vegetable protein (TVP) can all take on a meaty texture in meals like tacos, chili, or shepherd's pie.

Burgers and sausages: Black bean burgers, lentil burgers, portobello mushroom burgers, or veggie sausages are delicious choices.

Dairy:

Milk: As mentioned above, plant-based milks are great substitutes.

Cheese: Nutritional yeast adds a cheesy taste to dishes like pasta or popcorn. Cashew cheese or tofu scramble can replace ricotta in lasagna or breakfast scrambles.

Yogurt: Soy yogurt, coconut yogurt, or homemade cashew yogurt are creamy and delicious plant-based choices.

Eggs:

Binding: Flaxseed meal mixed with water makes a sticky consistency similar to an egg. Chia seeds can also be used as a required agent.

Scrambled eggs: Tofu scramble with turmeric for color is a classic vegan breakfast choice. Chickpea flour omelets (socca) are another clever swap.

Tips:

1. **Experiment with flavors:** Vegan cooking is all about discovering different textures and tastes. Don't be afraid to try with spices and herbs to create exciting flavor profiles.

2. **Embrace new ingredients:** Tempeh, seitan, and jackfruit might be new names, but they

can be amazing additions to your vegan menu. Research recipes and discover how to use them!

3. **Start with known dishes:** Make vegan versions of your favorite meals – vegan lasagna, mac and "cheese," or chili – to ease into the shift.

Simple Kitchen Tools for Effortless Vegan Cooking

You don't need a fancy kitchen to make great vegan food. Here are some simple tools that will come in handy:

- **Pots and pans:** A good set of pots and pans is necessary for sauteing, boiling, simmering, and stewing. Look for a range of sizes, including a large pot for pasta or soups, a medium saucepan for sauces and grains, and a frying pan for everyday cooking. Non-stick options make cleaning easy.

- **Sharp knives:** A good chef's knife is your best friend in the kitchen. It should feel comfortable in your hand and be able to handle a range of chopping tasks. A serrated knife is also handy for slicing bread or peppers.
- **Cutting board:** A sturdy cutting board will protect your countertops and make chopping

veggies safer. Opt for a large board to provide ample room

- **Mixing bowls:** You'll need a range of sizes for mixing ingredients, preparing batters, and tossing salads. Stainless steel or glass bowls are easy to clean and flexible.
- **Spatulas:** A rubber spatula for scraping bowls and a slotted spatula for flipping pancakes or burgers are necessary.
- *Measuring cups and spoons:* Accurate measurement ensures good results. Invest in a good set of measuring cups (dry and liquid) and spoons.
- **Blender or food processor:** These appliances are lifesavers

for making smoothies, pureeing sauces, grinding nuts, and chopping veggies. A handheld immersion blender is a space-saving choice that can handle many tasks.

- **Grater:** Freshly grated veggies and cheese (vegan cheese, of course!) add a burst of flavor and texture to dishes. Look for a grater with multiple sides for coarse and fine grinding.
- **Can opener and veggie peeler:** These simple tools make prepping ingredients a breeze.

Tips:

- **Invest in quality over quantity:** A few good quality tools will last you longer and work better than a collection of cheap ones.

- **Take care of your knives:** Keep your knives sharp for safety and ease of use. Learn right sharpening techniques or get them professionally sharpened.
- **Organize your tools:** Having your tools within easy reach makes cooking more efficient and fun.

Embrace the Journey!

With a well-stocked pantry, a few clever swaps, and some basic tools, you're ready to start on your delicious vegan adventure! Remember, cooking should be fun and artistic. Don't be afraid to explore, have fun, and most importantly, enjoy the delicious and nutritious meals you make in your plant-based kitchen!

PART 2: DELICIOUS MEALS IN MINUTES - FUELING YOUR DAY THE VEGAN WAY

You don't have to give up good eating just because your life is busy. This part will show you how to quickly make tasty vegan meals that are great for busy mornings, light lunches, and quick dinners during the week.

Breakfast on the Go (Smoothies, Bowls, and Quick Bites)

Even though mornings are busy, skipping breakfast makes you tired and more likely to eat unhealthy snacks. Here are some quick and easy vegan choices that will get you going:

Smoothies are an easy and quick way to get a lot of nutrients. For extra protein, mix your favorite plant-based milk with frozen fruits (like bananas, berries, and mango), leafy greens (like spinach and kale), nut butter, and chia seeds. Mix until smooth, then take a sip on your way out the door!

Tip:

Make the smoothie ingredients ahead of time and put them in the freezer in pre-measured amounts for easy access.

Breakfast Bowls: These customizable bowls are a fun and

filling way to start your day. If you want a base, try rolled oats with plant-based milk. If you want chopped veggies, try berries or melon. Top with your favorites like chopped nuts, seeds, shredded coconut, a drizzle of nut butter, or a spoonful of vegan yogurt. Tip: Keep a selection of chopped nuts, seeds, and dried fruits on hand for easy topping choices.

Quick Bites: Need something you can eat on the run? Here are some ideas:

Whole-wheat toast with mashed avocado or a dollop of hummus and chopped tomato.

A handful of almonds or walnuts with a chunk of fruit.

A pre-made vegan breakfast bar with whole grains, nuts, and dried fruit.

Tip:

Pack a small cooler bag with your breakfast and an ice pack if you have a longer journey.

Light and Satisfying Lunches (Salads, Wraps, and Soups)

Lunch should be about refueling your body for the afternoon. Here are some light yet filling vegan options:

Salads: Salads don't have to be boring! Layer a bed of leafy greens with a range of colorful vegetables, chopped nuts, seeds, and a flavorful vegan dressing. Add some protein with beans, lentils, tofu cubes, or tempeh.

Tip:

Prepare a big batch of cooked chickpeas or lentils on the weekend to have protein easily available for salads throughout the week.

Wraps: Wraps are a portable and customizable lunch choice. Spread a whole-wheat wrap with hummus, pesto, or vegan mayonnaise. Fill with chopped veggies, leafy greens, sliced avocado, and your protein of choice. Tip: Pre-chop veggies and store them in an airtight container for quick and easy wrap assembly.

Soups: Soups are a warm and nourishing lunch choice. Opt for lentil soup, minestrone with veggie "meatballs," or creamy tomato soup. Leftover soup can be quickly reheated for a quick lunch the next day.

Tip: Make a large pot of soup on the weekend and portion it out for work lunches. Freeze extra portions for a quick and convenient choice later.

Weeknight Dinners in 30 Minutes (One-Pot Wonders, Stir-fries, and Pastas)

Weeknights can be especially difficult when it comes to cooking. Here are some amazing and delightful vegan meals you can whip up in 30 minutes or less:

One-Pot Wonders: These easy meals minimize cleanup and increase flavor. Here are some ideas:

Stir-fry: Saute chopped veggies with tofu, tempeh, or seitan in a wok or large pan. Add your favorite stir-fry sauce and serve over brown rice or grain.

Curries: Curries are packed with taste and can be easily made vegan. Choose from chickpea curry, lentil curry, or a creamy coconut curry with veggies. Serve over rice or naan bread.

Pasta Primavera: Cook whole-wheat pasta according to package directions. While the pasta is cooking, saute a range of seasonal vegetables in olive oil. Toss everything together with a simple sauce of lemon juice, garlic, and herbs.

Tip: Chop veggies in advance and store them in an airtight container for quicker prep time.

Pasta Dishes: Pasta is a dinner staple, and it can easily be made vegan.

Tomato Pasta: Saute chopped onions and garlic, add canned crushed tomatoes, spices (Italian seasoning, red pepper flakes), and boil. Toss with cooked whole-wheat pasta and top with vegan parmesan cheese (made from nuts!)

Creamy Vegan Pasta: Blend wet cashews with nutritional yeast, lemon juice, and water for a creamy sauce. Toss

Tip: Cook a double batch of pasta and use the extras for lunch salads or another quick dinner later in the week.

General Tips for Quick and Easy Vegan Meals:

Plan your meals: Dedicate some time each week to plan your meals and make a grocery list. This will save you time and money at the store, and help you avoid unhealthy last-minute choices.

Prep in advance: Chopping vegetables, preparing grains, and cooking tofu or lentils in advance can greatly reduce your cooking time on busy weeknights.

Utilize leftovers: Leftovers can be a lifesaver! Repurpose leftovers into new recipes. For example, leftover roasted veggies can be added to pasta or stir-fries, or leftover cooked grains can be used in salads or breakfast bowls.

Embrace frozen vegetables: Frozen vegetables are a handy and affordable way to add variety and nutrients to your meals. They're often flash-frozen at peak ripeness and keep their vitamins and minerals.

Don't be afraid of shortcuts: There's no shame in using pre-made ingredients like pre-washed and chopped veggies, pre-cooked brown rice, or store-bought vegan sauces. These can save you important time in the kitchen.

Remember, cooking should be fun! With a little planning and these quick and easy recipes, you can whip up delicious and healthy vegan meals without spending hours in the kitchen. So, unleash your inner chef, accept the convenience factor, and enjoy the delicious world of plant-based cooking!

PART 3: PLANT-BASED COMFORT FOOD - SATISFYING YOUR CRAVINGS, VEGAN STYLE

Comfort food – those warm, familiar dishes that evoke a sense of nostalgia and pleasure. The good news? You don't have to give up your favorite comfort foods when going veggie! This section will show you how to make delicious vegan versions of classic dishes, hearty soups and stews, and decadent desserts, all without compromising on taste or comfort.

Vegan Takes on Classic Dishes (Burgers, Mac and "Cheese," and Curries)

Sometimes you just crave a basic dish. Here are some delicious vegan spins on your favorites:

Burgers: Vegan burgers are no longer a sad replacement!

Black Bean Burgers: Mashed black beans, chopped vegetables, and spices come together to make a hearty and flavorful patty. Grill, pan-fry, or bake your burgers and enjoy them on a whole-wheat bun with your favorite toppings.

Lentil Burgers: Lentils provide a great base for a juicy burger.

Combine cooked lentils with breadcrumbs, chopped veggies, and spices. Form into patties and cook as preferred.

Portobello Mushroom Burgers: Marinated portobello mushrooms make a meaty and satisfying burger alternative. Grill or pan-fry the mushrooms and pile them high with your favorite toppings on a warm bun.

Tip: Experiment with different flavorings in your veggie burgers. Add spices like cumin, chili powder, or smoked paprika for a smoky taste.

Mac and "Cheese": This classic comfort food gets a delicious veggie makeover. Here are two options:

Cashew Cheese Sauce: Soaked cashews blended with nutritional yeast, lemon juice, and spices make a creamy and cheesy sauce perfect for macaroni.

Nutritional Yeast Sauce: Nutritional yeast adds a cheesy taste to a simple sauce made with plant-based milk, flour, and spices.

Tip: Top your veggie mac and "cheese" with breadcrumbs for a crispy topping.

Curries: Curries are a fantastic way to discover a world of flavors.

Chickpea Curry: This hearty curry features chickpeas simmered in a flavorful coconut curry sauce with veggies like onions, peppers, and carrots. Serve over rice or naan bread.

Thai Curry: Explore different versions of Thai curries – red, green, or yellow – using vegetables like eggplant, bell peppers, and tofu. Serve with brown rice or rice noodles.

Tip: Adjust the spice level of your curries to your taste. Add a touch of cayenne pepper for a kick or make it mild with coconut milk.

Hearty and Warming Soups and Stews

There's nothing quite as comfortable as a warm bowl of soup or stew on a chilly day. These veggie options will leave you feeling satisfied and nourished:

Lentil Soup: This filling soup is packed with protein and fiber. Lentils are simmered with veggies, herbs, and spices for a flavorful and satisfying meal.

Minestrone Soup: This classic Italian soup gets a vegan makeover with vegetable "meatballs" made from beans or tempeh. Packed with veggies and pasta, it's a complete meal in a bowl.

Split Pea Soup: Split peas simmered with vegetables and flavorful spices like smoked paprika and thyme make a soul-warming and satisfying soup.

Chickpea Stew with Coconut Milk: This stew includes chickpeas, vegetables, and a creamy coconut milk broth. Serve with rice for a full meal.

Tip: Cook a big pot of soup or stew on the weekend and portion it out for quick and easy meals throughout the week.

Sweet Treats to Satisfy (sweets without the Dairy)

Who says you can't indulge in delicious sweets while vegan? Here are some great dairy-free treats:

Fruit Crumble: Top your favorite seasonal fruits with a crumble covering made from rolled oats, nuts, and spices. Bake until golden brown and enjoy a warm and cozy dessert.

Chocolate Avocado Mousse: This delicious mousse is surprisingly easy to make. Blend ripe avocado with cocoa powder, maple syrup, and plant-based milk for a rich and creamy treat.

Baked Apples: Baked apples filled with chopped nuts, raisins, and a touch of cinnamon are a healthy and delicious dessert. Top with a scoop of vegan ice cream for an extra treat.

Vegan Chocolate Chip Cookies: Classic chocolate chip cookies can be easily made vegan. Use vegan butter and chocolate chips, and you'll never miss the dairy!

Tip: Explore the world of plant-based milks like almond milk, oat milk, or coconut milk for baking. Each adds a slightly different taste profile to your desserts.

General Tips for Comfort Food:

Don't be afraid of good fats: Healthy fats like avocados, nuts, and seeds add richness and creaminess to vegan comfort food recipes. Embrace them for a satisfying taste and texture.

Spice it up!: Spices and herbs play a crucial role in creating depth of flavor in vegan food. Experiment with different combinations like smoked paprika and cumin for a smoky depth, or curry powder and turmeric for a warm Indian-inspired taste.

Embrace leftovers: Leftover soups, stews, and curries can be quickly transformed into other dishes. Use extra chickpea curry in a wrap for lunch, or repurpose leftover lentil soup into a shepherd's pie with mashed potatoes.

Don't forget the presentation: Even simple meals can be made visually appealing with a little effort. Plate your food carefully, garnish with fresh herbs, and enjoy the satisfaction of a delicious and healthy meal you made yourself.

The Joy of Plant-Based Comfort Food

Vegan comfort food isn't about deprivation, it's about enjoying delicious plant-based ingredients and making dishes that nourish your body and soul. These recipes are just a starting point – experiment, have fun, and find the endless possibilities of vegan comfort food! So grab your favorite vegetables, spices, and a dash of imagination, and get ready to indulge in a world of flavorful and satisfying vegan comfort food.

Part 4: Living A Healthy Vegan Lifestyle - Making Veganism Work For You

Going vegan is a fantastic way to boost your health and explore a delicious world of plant-based food. But let's face it, life can get busy, and navigating a new way of eating can seem daunting. This section will equip you with practical tips for meal planning, eating out vegan, and creating a balanced vegan plate, making your vegan journey smooth and enjoyable.

Meal Planning for Busy Weeks

Planning your meals ahead of time is key to success, especially when life gets hectic. Here's how to make meal planning a breeze:

- **Dedicate some time each week:** Set aside 30 minutes to plan your meals for the week. Browse cookbooks, online resources, or this book for inspiration!
- **Consider your schedule:** Plan quick and easy meals for busy days and more elaborate dishes for when you have more time.
- **Create a grocery list:** Based on your meal plan, create a detailed grocery list to avoid impulse purchases at the store.

- **Utilize leftovers:** Plan meals that can be repurposed for leftovers. Leftover roasted vegetables can be added to salads or stir-fries, and leftover cooked grains can be used in breakfast bowls or veggie burgers.

Tips:

- **Cook in bulk:** If you have time on the weekend, cook a double batch of a dish like lentil soup or chili. Portion it out for quick and easy meals throughout the week.
- **Prep in advance:** Chopping vegetables, prepping grains, and

cooking tofu or lentils in advance can significantly reduce your cooking time on busy weeknights.

- **Utilize frozen vegetables:** Frozen vegetables are a lifesaver! They're affordable, convenient, and packed with nutrients.

Simple Tips for Eating Out Vegan

Eating out doesn't have to be a challenge when you're vegan. Here are some tips to navigate restaurants and social gatherings with ease:

- **Research the menu beforehand:** Many restaurants offer vegan options these days. Look at their menu online or call ahead to inquire about vegan possibilities.

- **Don't be afraid to ask questions:** If the menu descriptions aren't clear, politely ask your server about vegan options. They can often modify dishes to be vegan by omitting cheese or dairy-based sauces.

- **Popular Vegan Restaurant Choices:** Here are some restaurants that typically have vegan options:

- **Asian cuisine:** Many Thai, Indian, and Vietnamese restaurants offer naturally vegan dishes like curries, stir-fries, and noodle soups. Just be mindful of fish sauce in some dishes.
- **Mediterranean cuisine:** Falafel wraps, hummus plates, and lentil salads are all delicious vegan options found in many Mediterranean restaurants.
- **Mexican cuisine:** Opt for bean burritos, fajitas with vegetables and beans, or

ask for veggie tacos without
cheese or sour cream.

Tips:

- **Bring your own snacks:** If
  you're unsure about vegan
  options at a gathering, pack a
  healthy and filling snack like
  nuts, fruits, or a homemade
  energy bar.
- **Offer to bring a dish:** If you're
  going to a potluck or social
  gathering, volunteer to bring a
  vegan dish to share. It's a great
  way to introduce people to
  delicious plant-based food.

Building a Balanced Vegan Plate (Nutrients Made Easy)

Eating a balanced vegan diet ensures you get all the essential nutrients your body needs. Here's what to consider for a balanced vegan plate:

- **Grains:** Choose a variety of whole grains like brown rice, quinoa, oats, whole-wheat bread, and pasta. Whole grains provide sustained energy and fiber.
- **Vegetables:** Fill half your plate with a colorful array of vegetables. Aim for a variety of colors and textures for a range of vitamins and minerals.

- **Fruits:** Include fruits in your diet for essential vitamins, minerals, and antioxidants.
- **Protein:** While you don't need to worry about complete proteins at every meal, aim to include a variety of protein sources throughout the day. Beans, lentils, tofu, tempeh, nuts, and seeds are all excellent sources of plant-based protein.
- **Healthy Fats:** Healthy fats like avocados, nuts, seeds, and olive oil are essential for satiety and nutrient absorption. Include them in moderation in your meals.

Tips:

- **Don't be afraid of supplements:** Vitamin B12 is essential, and it's not readily available in plant-based foods. Consider taking a B12 supplement to ensure you're getting enough.
- **Read food labels:** Pay attention to fortified foods like plant-based milks that are often enriched with calcium and vitamin D.
- **Listen to your body:** Eat when you're hungry and stop when you're satisfied.

Embrace the Journey!

Living a healthy vegan lifestyle is not about restriction, it's about embracing delicious and nutritious plant-based foods. With a little planning and these tips, you can navigate your vegan journey with ease. Remember, this is a process, so be kind to yourself, have fun exploring new flavors and recipes, and celebrate your progress along the way!

Additional Resources:

- **Online Resources:** There are countless websites and blogs dedicated to vegan recipes, meal planning tips, and general vegan living advice. Explore and find resources that resonate with you.

- **Vegan Cookbooks:** Invest in a good vegan cookbook or two. They'll provide you with endless recipe inspiration and guidance.
- **Vegan Community:** Connect with other vegans online or in your local community. Sharing experiences, tips, and recipes can be a source of support and motivation.

Final Thoughts

Making the switch to a vegan lifestyle can be an incredibly rewarding experience. You'll not only be nourishing your body with delicious and healthy plant-based foods, but you'll also be contributing to a more sustainable planet. With the information and resources in this book, you're well on your way to embracing a happier, healthier, and more compassionate you!

Let's get cooking! This book is your guide to exploring the delicious world of vegan food. With easy-to-follow recipes, practical tips, and helpful information, you'll be whipping up amazing vegan meals in no time. So, turn the page, unleash your inner chef, and embark on a delicious and rewarding vegan adventure!

CONCLUSION: THE JOY OF SIMPLE VEGAN COOKING - A DELICIOUS AND REWARDING JOURNEY AWAITS!

Congratulations! You've reached the end of this exploration into the world of vegan cooking. Hopefully, you're feeling inspired and excited to create delicious and nutritious plant-based meals in your own kitchen. Remember, vegan cooking doesn't have to be complicated or time-consuming. Here's a final recap to solidify the joy and simplicity of vegan cuisine:

The Joy of Simple Vegan Cooking

Vegan cooking offers a wealth of benefits:

- **Delicious and Satisfying Food:** Plant-based meals can be incredibly flavorful and satisfying. Experiment with spices, herbs, and global cuisines to discover your favorites.
- **Enhanced Health and Well-being:** Vegan foods are packed with vitamins, minerals, fiber, and healthy fats, contributing to a healthier you.
- **Sustainable Living:** Choosing plant-based meals has a lower environmental impact compared to animal agriculture.

Tips for Enjoying the Process:

- **Don't be afraid to experiment:** Step outside your comfort zone and try new ingredients, recipes, and flavors. The world of vegan cuisine is vast and exciting!
- **Make it fun:** Cooking should be a joyful experience. Put on some music, grab a friend to help, and enjoy the process of creating something delicious.
- **Celebrate your successes:** Take pride in the meals you create. Savor the flavors and celebrate the healthy choices you're making.

Resources and Inspiration for Your Vegan Journey

Here are some resources to keep you motivated and inspired as you continue your vegan journey:

- **Online Resources:** The internet is a treasure trove of vegan resources. Explore websites and blogs dedicated to vegan recipes, meal planning, and general vegan living advice. Find reliable sources that resonate with your style and preferences.
- **Vegan Cookbooks:** Invest in a couple of good vegan cookbooks that offer diverse recipes and cooking techniques. These can be your go-to guides for inspiration and new ideas.

- **Vegan Community:** Connect with other vegans! Join online communities, follow vegan social media influencers, or find local vegan groups. Sharing experiences, tips, and recipes can be a valuable source of support and motivation.
- **Learn as you go:** The world of vegan cooking is constantly evolving. Stay curious, read articles about nutrition and plant-based ingredients, and keep learning and expanding your knowledge.

Final Thoughts:

Vegan cooking isn't about deprivation, it's about exploration and discovery. You'll find a whole new world of flavors, textures, and ingredients waiting to be explored. Embrace the process, have fun, and enjoy the delicious journey towards a healthier, happier, and more compassionate you!

Bonus Tip: Keep a notebook handy to jot down recipe ideas, adjustments you make to existing recipes, and your own culinary creations. This personal library will become a valuable resource and a testament to your growing expertise in vegan cooking!

With the tools and knowledge you've gained from this book, you're well on your way to becoming a confident vegan chef. So grab your favorite vegetables, spices, and a dash of creativity, and get cooking! Your taste buds and your body will thank you.

Acknowledgements: A Culinary Journey of Gratitude

In closing this exploration of the vibrant world of vegan cooking, a deep sense of gratitude washes over me. This book wouldn't exist without the countless people and experiences that have shaped my passion for plant-based cuisine.

Firstly, a heartfelt thank you goes out to my family and friends. Their unwavering support throughout my vegan journey has been invaluable. Their willingness to sample my culinary experiments, both successful and…well, let's just say "interesting," has been a constant source of encouragement. Their genuine curiosity about vegan food and their open-mindedness in trying new dishes motivated me to keep exploring and perfecting my skills.

A special shout-out goes to [Name of specific friend or family member]. Their [specific positive quality or action related to vegan food] truly opened my eyes to the possibilities of plant-based cuisine. Remember that time we [share a specific memory of a positive vegan food experience with this person]? That experience sparked a fire in me, inspiring me to delve deeper into the world of vegan flavors.

Secondly, I owe a debt of gratitude to the incredible vegan chefs, bloggers, and cookbook authors who have generously shared their knowledge and creativity. Their [mention specific resources like cookbooks, websites, or social media channels] became my launchpad, providing inspiration and guidance as I embarked on my vegan cooking journey. Poring over their recipes, learning from their techniques, and witnessing their passion for plant-based food ignited a spark in me.

Thirdly, a big thank you goes out to the entire vegan community. Connecting with other like-minded individuals online and in local groups has been a source of immense support and motivation. Sharing recipes, tips, and experiences has fostered a sense of camaraderie and belonging. The knowledge that I'm not alone in this journey, that there's a whole community of people passionate about delicious and healthy vegan food, has been incredibly inspiring.

Finally, a deep thank you goes out to you, the reader. Your decision to pick up this book speaks volumes about your curiosity and open-mindedness towards plant-based cooking. Whether you're a seasoned vegan looking for new culinary adventures or someone just starting to explore the world of vegan food, I hope this book serves as a valuable resource and a springboard for your own culinary discoveries.

As I reflect on the journey that led to this book, a few key takeaways surface – lessons learned that I want to share with you:

- **Embrace the learning process:** Don't be afraid to experiment and make mistakes in the kitchen. Those "oops" moments, while frustrating at times, often lead to unexpected discoveries and new culinary creations.
- **Don't be afraid to get creative:** Vegan cooking offers a vast canvas for your creativity. Substitute, swap, and experiment with flavors and ingredients to

find dishes that tantalize your taste buds.

- **The power of community:** Connecting with other vegans can be an invaluable source of support and inspiration. Share your knowledge, learn from others, and celebrate your culinary successes together.

- **Most importantly, have fun!** Cooking should be a joyful experience. So, put on some music, grab a friend to help, laugh off any mishaps, and savor the delicious creations you bring to life.

This book is more than just a collection of recipes; it's an invitation to explore the boundless possibilities of vegan cooking. With a little practice, creativity, and the support of this wonderful vegan community, you too can unlock a world of delicious and healthy plant-based meals.

So, grab your favorite vegetables, spices, and a dash of curiosity, and get cooking! Your taste buds and your body will thank you.

With heartfelt gratitude,

MARYANN D. LANG